DR SE_____ ___ ___
ALL DISEASES

The step by step proven natural treatment for diseases such as HIV, AIDs, STDs, herpes, Cancer, Diabetes, herpes, erectile dysfunction. arthritis, kidney/liver diseases and other chronic diseases.

By **George J. Gibbs**

TABLE OF CONTENTS

CHAPTER 1

INTRODUCTION

The late Dr. Sebi created the Dr. Sebi diet, also known as the Dr. The Sebi alkaline diet is a plant-based diet. By removing harmful waste from your body, which is supposedly performed by alkalizing your blood, it is stated to renew your cells.

The diet includes a broad list of supplements in addition to a small number of permitted foods.

You might, however, question whether its claims are supported by scientific data and whether it's healthful.

What Exactly Is This Dr Sebi Diet

This diet was created by self-taught herbalist Alfredo Darrington Bowman, often known as Dr. Dr. Sebi's philosophy is based on African Bio-Mineral Balance.. Sebi was neither a medical doctor nor a PhD, despite his name.

He created this diet for anyone who wants to improve their general health, organically treat or prevent disease, and avoid using traditional Western medicine.

Dr. Sebi claims that any part of your body where mucus builds up might lead to sickness. He asserted that diabetes is brought on by an abundance of mucus in the pancreas, whereas pneumonia is brought on by a buildup of mucus in the lungs.

He argued that diseases start when your body becomes overly acidic and cannot thrive in an alkaline environment. His diet and expensive, proprietary supplements promise to detoxify your sick body and return it to its original alkaline state.

Initially, Dr. Sebi asserted that this diet could treat diseases like lupus, leukemia, sickle cell disease, and AIDS. However, he was told to stop making them after a 1993 lawsuit.

The diet consists of a certain set of permitted grains, nuts, seeds, fruits, vegetables, oils, and herbs. The Dr. Sebi diet is regarded as a vegan diet because animal products are not allowed.

According to Sebi, you must adhere to the diet religiously for the rest of your life if you want your body to repair itself.

Dr. Sebi's diet, according to many testimonies, has improved chromic disorders.

SUMMARY

The Dr. Sebi diet places an emphasis on foods and supplements that are claimed to cause your body to become more alkaline, hence reducing disease-causing mucus. But these claims haven't been supported by any studies.

CHAPTER 2

HOW TO GET AN ALKALINE BODY: A STEP-BY-STEP GUIDE?

Here are some things to know and do to help your body reach that alkaline state:

In general terms, what does it mean to eat in an alkaline manner?

There are a few different names for the alkaline diet, but the most common ones are the acid-alkaline diet and the alkaline ash diet.

The theory behind it is that you can alter your body's pH (a measure of how acidic or alkaline it is) through what you eat.

Your metabolism, the process by which food is converted into energy, has been compared to fire. The solid material in both cases must undergo a chemical reaction in order to be dissolved.

In contrast, the chemical reactions inside your body are gradual and carefully controlled.

After a fire has burned something down, it leaves behind a charred ash. Metabolic waste is the discarded "ash" from the food you eat.

It's possible that the metabolic waste products are pH-neutral, acidic, or alkaline. The acidity of your body, proponents of this diet claim, can be changed directly by metabolic waste.

The acidity of the blood is increased when foods high in ash are consumed. Consuming foods that result in alkaline ash causes your blood to become more alkaline.

According to the acid-ash hypothesis, consuming alkaline ash is protective while consuming acidic ash increases your susceptibility to disease.

If you "alkalize" your diet and adopt a more acidic lifestyle, you may see an improvement in your health.

Producing an acidic ash from foods high in protein, phosphate, or sulfur, and a basic ash from foods high in calcium, magnesium, or potassium.

Different food groups are considered neutral, alkaline, or acidic, respectively.

Acidic foods include animal products, seafood, eggs, cereals, and alcohol.

Natural sources of sugars, fats, and carbs

Naturally occurring alkaline foods include those found in the plant kingdom.

According to advocates of the alkaline diet, the ash that remains after food is burned has a direct effect on the acidity or alkalinity of the body.

The pH levels in your body are stable.

Having a firm grasp on pH is essential when discussing the alkaline diet.

pH is a scale used to indicate how acidic or basic a substance is.

pH scale values can be anywhere from zero to fourteen.

Range: 7.0 to 14.0 for alkaline; 0.0 to 6.9 for acidic; 7.0 is neutral.

Many proponents of this diet stress the importance of monitoring urine pH to ensure that it remains above 7 and is not acidic (below 7).

Bear in mind that your body's pH fluctuates greatly. Certain locations are more acidic while others are more alkaline, but the overall acidity level is not fixed.

The hydrochloric acid in your stomach lowers its pH to a very acidic 2–3.5. In order to break down food, this acidity is required.

However, the pH of human blood is always between 7.36 and 7.44, making it somewhat alkaline.

An abnormal blood pH balance can be dangerous if left untreated.

However, this is something that only happens under very particular medical conditions, such as diabetic ketoacidosis, malnutrition, or excessive alcohol intake.

SYNOPSIS The acidity or alkalinity of a substance can be measured using the pH scale. When compared to the extreme acidity of stomach acid, blood's mild alkalinity is illustrative.

Food impacts urine pH, not blood.

The maintenance of good health depends on the constancy of the blood's pH.

If it was abnormally low, your cells would stop working, and you would die quickly if you weren't treated.

Therefore, your body adapts a wide range of sophisticated systems for keeping the pH balance in check. This is what is meant by the term "acid-base homeostasis."

Although some variations within the normal range are possible, it is highly unlikely that a healthy person's blood pH would be affected by their diet.

However, the pH of your urine can be affected by what you eat, though the effects will be different for everyone.

Urine acid excretion is an important physiological mechanism for maintaining a healthy blood pH.

Your urine will become more acidic as your body eliminates the metabolic waste from eating a huge steak a few hours later.

Therefore, urine pH is not an adequate indicator of either overall health or body pH. Many factors can influence it, not just the food you eat.

SUMMARY

The blood's acidity or alkalinity is strictly regulated by your body. In healthy people, dietary changes don't significantly affect blood pH but can affect the pH of urine.

Foods high in uric acid and the risk of osteoporosis

Osteoporosis, a degenerative bone disease, is characterized by a decrease in bone mineral content.

Postmenopausal women are at a higher risk for developing this condition, which increases their fragility and thus their likelihood of breaking a bone.

Many advocates of the alkaline diet claim that the body uses calcium and other alkaline minerals from the bones to neutralize the acid produced by the digestion of acidic meals.

According to this theory, acid-producing foods like the standard Western diet cause bones to become weaker and less dense.

However, this view ignores the significance of the kidneys in neutralizing acids and maintaining a healthy body pH.

The kidneys produce bicarbonate ions, which neutralize acids in the blood, allowing the body to carefully manage blood pH.

Your body's respiratory system plays a role in controlling blood pH. When bicarbonate ions from the kidneys bond to acids in the blood, you exhale carbon dioxide and urinate water.

One of the main causes of osteoporosis is the loss of the collagen-rich protein from bone, which is not taken into consideration by the acid-ash hypothesis.

Loss of collagen is paradoxically linked to deficiencies in two acids: orthosilicic acid and ascorbic acid, or vitamin C.

Keep in mind that research linking dietary acid to bone density or fracture risk is inconclusive. While many observational studies have shown no connection, others have found one.

It has been established through more credible clinical studies that acid-

There is zero correlation between calcium intake and blood levels.

Bone health is enhanced by these diets because they increase calcium absorption and stimulate the IGF-1 hormone, which aids in muscle and bone regeneration.

Therefore, a high-protein diet that also includes acid-producing foods is likely associated with better bone health.

CONCLUSION Despite some contradictory evidence, the vast majority of studies do not support the claim that acid-forming foods are bad for your bones. Even though protein is an acidic food, it nevertheless seems to have benefits.

CHAPTER 3:

ACIDITY AND THE RISK OF CANCER

Since cancer can only survive in an acidic environment, many individuals believe an alkaline diet can treat or even cure cancer.

However, extensive research into the possible link between diet-induced acidosis (or dietary-caused increases in blood acidity) and cancer found no such correlation.

To begin, there is negligible if any impact on blood pH from eating.

The second is that cancer cells are not only present in acidic environments, even if you think that eating may drastically alter the pH of blood or other organs.

Truth be told, cancer forms in slightly alkaline (pH 7.4) healthy bodily tissue. A large number of experiments have shown that an alkaline medium is optimal for growing cancer cells.

Moreover, tumors not only flourish in acidic environments, but they also manufacture the acidity themselves. It is the cancer cells themselves that create an acidic environment, not the environment itself.

TIPS FOR STAYING ON THE DR. SEBI DIET

CHAPTER 4
THE RULES OF THE DR. SEBI DIET

The rules of the Dr. Sebi diet are extremely strict.:

First and foremost, only eat what is listed in the food pyramid.

Second rule: Drink a full gallon (3.8 liters) of water every day.

The third rule is to take Dr. Sebi's vitamins an hour before taking any prescription drugs.

No animal products are allowed, according to Rule 4. \s5. There will be no booze allowed.

• Don't eat any wheat products and stick to the "natural-growing grains" recommended in the book, which is rule number six.

Do not use a microwave if you don't want to "kill" your food.

When in doubt, rule 8 states that you should not eat canned or seedless fruit.

Nutrient requirements and preferences are not specified. This diet is low in protein since it disallows several common sources. Protein is an important nutrient because it helps maintain strong muscles, smooth skin, and flexible joints.

In addition, you must purchase Dr. Sebi's "cell food" supplements, which are said to purge toxins from the body's cells and restore their vitality.

No recommended vitamins or minerals are mentioned. Instead, you should make a purchase of a health supplement that specifically addresses your needs.

To give just one example, the "Bio Ferro" capsules claim to alleviate liver issues, cleanse the blood, fortify the immune system, promote weight loss, aid in digestion, and enhance general health.

Because of the absence of a comprehensive list of nutrients and their quantities, determining if the supplements will satisfy your daily needs can be difficult.

SUMMARY

The Dr. Sebi diet has eight primary tenets that must be followed. Their main tenets include a lack of animal products, a rejection of processed foods, and the use of targeted nutritional aids.

CHAPTER 5

CONSIDERABLE DR. SEBI DIET WEIGHT LOSS OPPORTUNITIES IN

The goal of Dr. Sebi's diet isn't weight loss, although it can be accomplished with dedication.

The diet discourages a Western diet that is high in ultra-processed foods that are high in salt, sugar, fat, and calories.

As an alternative, it promotes a diet rich in unprocessed plant foods. The prevalence of obesity and cardiovascular disease are both reduced on plant-based diets compared to Western diets.

An analysis of a 12-month study involving 65 people found that those who consumed an unlimited supply of whole foods and low-fat plant-based meals lost significantly more weight than those who did not.

Six months into the diet, the participants lost an average of 26.6 pounds (12.1 kg), while the controls lost only 3.5 pounds (1.7 kg) (1.6 kg).

Most of the foods on this diet are low in calories, with the exception of oils, nuts, seeds, avocados, and some oils. Therefore, it is unlikely that eating a lot of permitted foods would result in excessive calorie consumption and subsequent weight gain.

However, extremely low-calorie diets are notoriously difficult to maintain over the long term. Following one of these diets usually ends in weight gain when a regular eating schedule is resumed.

Because it doesn't specify amounts, it's tough to tell if this diet will provide enough calories for sustainable weight loss.

SYNOPSIS Though it's not its primary purpose, the Dr. Sebi diet is low in calories and limits processed foods. Therefore, if you follow this diet plan, you may experience some weight loss.

OPTIONS IN DR. SEBI'S DIET

One benefit of the Dr. Sebi diet is that it places a premium on plant-based foods.

Fruits and vegetables are highly recommended on this diet due to their abundance of beneficial fiber, vitamins, minerals, and other plant-based substances. Fruit and vegetable-rich diets have been associated with reduced oxidative stress and inflammation, as well as protection from several diseases.

Those who consumed seven or more servings of fruits and vegetables per day had a 25% lower risk of cardiovascular disease and a 31% lower risk of cancer, according to a study of 65,226 people.

On top of that, most people don't eat enough vegetables and fruits. One study found that only 9.3% of people and 12.2% of people, respectively, met the recommendations for fruit and vegetables.

In addition, Dr. Sebi recommends consuming high-fiber whole grains and healthy fats like nuts, seeds, and plant oils. Some foods have been linked to a reduced risk of developing heart disease.

In conclusion, research has shown that diets low in ultra-processed foods have positive effects on health.

SUMMARY

Diets like Dr. Sebi's, which emphasize nutrient-dense fruits and vegetables, whole grains, and healthy fats, have been shown to reduce inflammation, cancer, and heart disease risk.

CHAPTER 7

CONS CONCERNING THE DR. SEBI DIET

Please keep in mind that there are many drawbacks to this diet.

restrictive to the extreme

A major drawback of Dr. Sebi's diet is that it prohibits eating many common foods. These include all animal products, wheat, beans, lentils, and many varieties of vegetables and fruits.

It is so strict that only certain types of fruit are allowed. For instance, you can only use cherry or plum tomatoes, but not beefsteak or Roma varieties.

In addition, since it disparages foods that aren't included in its nutrition guide, following such a stringent diet may not be enjoyable and may lead to a negative connection with food.

This diet also encourages other unhealthy behaviors, such as taking supplements just to stay full. This statement promotes unhealthy eating habits, as supplements do not provide many calories.

poor in protein and other essential nutrients.

When followed, Dr. Sebi's nutritional recommendations can be a great way to get the nutrients your body needs.

Protein is essential for many bodily functions, including cell repair, muscle growth, hormone and enzyme production, and skin and hair health, but none of the permitted meals provide adequate amounts.

Even the few nuts that are permitted (walnuts, Brazil nuts, sesame seeds, and hemp seeds) aren't very high in protein. 1/4 cup (25 grams) of walnuts and 3 tablespoons (30 grams) of hemp seeds, for example, each contain 4 and 9 grams of protein, respectively. To meet your daily protein needs from these foods, you would need to eat extremely large quantities.

Beta carotene, potassium, vitamins C and E, and other antioxidants are plentiful in the foods included in this diet, but iron, calcium, omega-3 fatty acids, and vitamins D and B12 are often in short supply, causing concern for those who follow a plant-based diet.

Some of the supplement components are secret, according to the Dr. Sebi diet website. Having no idea which nutrients you're getting or how much of them is worrisome because it makes it impossible to know if you'll meet your daily nutrient needs.

not backed by scientific evidence

One of the major problems is that Dr. Sebi's nutrition strategy has no scientific backing.

You can control your body's acid production, the diet says, thanks to the foods and supplements it recommends. However, because the human body strictly regulates the acid-base balance to keep blood pH values between 7.36 and

7.44, people tend to become slightly alkaline as they age.

Blood pH outside of this range is extremely unusual but is possible in extreme cases like diabetic ketoacidosis. It could be fatal if someone doesn't get help fast.

Finally, studies have shown that diet can slightly and temporarily affect urine pH but not blood pH. And so, following Dr. Sebi's diet won't make your body more alkaline (21).

SUMMARY

Diets like Dr. Sebi's may help you lose weight, but they're unhealthy and lacking in essential nutrients like protein, omega-3 fatty acids, iron, calcium, vitamin D, and vitamin B12. The body's ability to maintain a healthy blood pH is also disregarded.

CHAPTER 8:

HOW SAFE IS THE DR. SEBI DIET?

The restricted nature of Dr. Sebi's diet means that he's missing out on a lot of nutrients. Your body may be able to make it through a short period of time on this diet, but it's not sustainable or healthy in the long run. To add insult to injury, it's unlikely that any dietary regimen could cause your blood pH to rise.

Following this diet for more than a few weeks may leave you vulnerable to micronutrient shortages and malnutrition due to the exclusion of foods rich in protein, omega-3 fatty acids, calcium, iron, vitamin D, and vitamin B12.

People with mineral deficiencies may have a harder time than others, especially those who already have health issues like osteoporosis, osteopenia, or iron deficiency anemia. The Dr. Sebi diet could potentially exacerbate existing conditions because it lacks certain essential micronutrients.

Not getting enough vitamin B12 can lead to pernicious anemia, which manifests with fatigue, memory loss, difficulty breathing, tingling in the hands and feet, and a raw, red tongue.

This diet is extremely harmful for certain people groups, including those who have or currently suffer from eating disorders and those who are expecting a child.

Talking to a doctor or registered dietitian before beginning this diet is recommended for anyone with kidney disease.

CONCLUSION Malnutrition may occur with prolonged Dr. Sebi diet use. This diet should be completely avoided during pregnancy and by anyone with a history of eating disorders.

FOODS APPROPRIATE FOR THE DR. SEBI DIET (CHAPTER 9)

Dr. Sebi's nutritional guide prohibits eating foods like:

Fruits include: apples, cantaloupe, currants, dates, figs, elderberries, papayas, berries, peaches, soft jelly coconuts, seeded key limes, mangoes, prickly pears, seeded melons, Latin or West Indies soursop, and tamarind. Nuts, seeds, and vegetables include: Brazil nuts, hemp seeds, raw sesame seeds, raw tahini butter, and walnuts. Other vegetables include bell peppers, cactus flowers, chickpeas, cucumbers, dandelion greens, and a variety of nuts and seeds.

Avocado oil, unrefined coconut oil, grape seed oil, hemp seed oil, unrefined olive oil, and sesame oil are all examples of oils.

• Some examples of herbal teas include elderberry, chamomile, fennel, tila, burdock, ginger, and raspberry.

• Spices like achiote, cayenne, habanero, tarragon, onion powder, sage, oregano, basil, cloves, bay leaf, dill, sweet basil, kosher salt, thyme, granulated seaweed, pure agave syrup, and dates.

You can alternate between sips of tea and water.

Furthermore, you may eat grains like pasta, cereal, bread, and flour. Nonetheless, you can't eat anything that calls for leavening with yeast or baking soda.

Can you recommend some alkaline-rich foods?

Since the foods you eat have a negligible effect on your blood's pH, there is no medical reason to limit yourself to the ones we've already listed.

Alkaline-inducing foods are plentiful, and they mainly consist of fruits, vegetables, nuts, and whole grains. The combination of these foods has been shown to extend life and improve health.

As a result, there are a great many upsides to eating more plant foods. Basically, Dr. Sebi's list isn't exhaustive of the foods that are good for you.

That's why it's important to consider including the following foods in your diet:

There were also fresh coconuts and kiwis in addition to the usual fare of potatoes, Swiss chard, Brussels sprouts, broccoli, iceberg lettuce, and cauliflower. Beans and lentils fell into the category of legumes.

Among the protein options is tofu.

SUMMARY

The Dr. Sebi diet allows for a very small selection of foods. Yet, a healthy diet should include a wide range of plant-based options.

Things to Avoid While Following the Dr. Sebi Diet

Canned fruits and vegetables, fruit without their seeds, and anything else not included in Dr. Sebi's nutrition guide are strictly prohibited.

Included are a wide variety of dairy, meat, and soy products.

foods that have been fortified, such as those sold by restaurants or delivered via food services; alcoholic beverages •

Yeast and yeast-based products • wheat Yeast or baking powder; sugar (other than date sugar and agave syrup)

Additionally, many types of grains, fruits, vegetables, nuts, and seeds are off-limits.

The diet eliminates or severely limits processed foods, animal products, and foods made with leavening agents. Some vegetables, grains, nuts, and seeds are off-limits as well.

Recipes and a menu sample

In this three-day Dr. Sebi diet plan example, we will examine a sample menu.

Breakfast on Day 1: two spelt and banana pancakes drizzled with agave syrup.

Lunch is an olive oil and basil-dressed kale salad with tomatoes, onions, avocado, dandelion greens, and chickpeas. Snack: a green juice smoothie with cucumbers, kale, apples, and ginger, measuring 1 cup (240 mL).

For dinner, we'll have vegetables in a stir-fry with some wild rice.

On the second day, have a smoothie for breakfast made with water, hemp seeds, bananas, and strawberries; bake blueberry muffins using blueberries, coconut milk, agave syrup, sea salt, oil, teff, and spelt flour; and top a homemade pizza with your preferred vegetables and Brazil nut cheese.

Chickpea burgers with spelt flour flatbread, tomato, onion, and kale will be tonight's supper. Tahini spread on rye bread with red pepper slices on the side.

On the third day, for breakfast, have some cooked quinoa with peaches, agave syrup, and unsweetened coconut milk.

Spelt pasta salad with key lime dressing, olive oil, and diced vegetables will be served for lunch. Mango, banana, and unsweetened coconut milk will be blended into a smoothie and served as a snack.

• Prepare a hearty vegetable soup with powdered seaweed, kale, onions, mushrooms, red bell peppers, and red wine for supper.

The primary focus of this example menu is on the permitted components listed in the diet's nutritional guidance. Fruits and vegetables take center stage in this diet, while other food groups are only represented in very small amounts.

THE ENDING

Dr. Sebi's diet recommends eating raw, organic plant-based foods.

Although it has the potential to aid in weight loss, it is extremely restrictive, lacks in certain nutrients, is reliant on the creator's expensive supplements, and makes unsubstantiated claims about putting your body into an alkaline state.

If you want to adopt a more plant-based eating pattern, there are many other healthy diets that are more flexible and long-lasting.

Made in the USA
Coppell, TX
08 July 2023

18805115R00020